Introduction

Thank you for choosing this book. If you are suffering from heart palpitations or arrhythmia, I hope to make this worth your while by sharing my own experiences of what worked and didn't work, and maybe even give you some concepts that will help you in your own journey. This book is written for people who have been to the doctor, had all the tests, and like myself, have been cleared of any "serious" medical condition, and told that they have premature atrial contractions (PACs), premature ventricular contractions (PVCs) or supraventricular tachycardia (SVT). I had all three, and this book is about how to manage or - dare I say it - cure these conditions.

First of all, I am not a doctor, but I have talked to plenty of them. If you are like most people who suffer from these "benign" arrhythmias, you have been told by every doctor that they are really harmless and nothing to worry about. While this may be true (once again, you need to get those tests to find out), for many of us, that doesn't change the sickening feeling of coping with these conditions every day. We are curious to learn more about these conditions and what triggers them, and in the case of ectopic beats (PACs and PVCs), the doctors seem to know next to nothing. We cast about for answers, Googling until our fingers are numb, and we end up buying dietary supplements by the truckload, possibly to little or no benefit.

Before we go any further, a brief introduction of myself. I'm a 32 year old male, 5' 9", 145 pounds. I've always considered myself a healthy person with a healthful diet, involved in sports when I was younger and with a job that keeps me relatively physically active. So why was I regularly experiencing the sensation that my heart had stopped beating for a moment, then restarted again with a "whomp" a moment later? I'll get to that soon enough.

When I was 17, I was walking around outside on my high school campus when my foot landed a little heavily on the ground, and all of a sudden I had the sensation that my heart was fluttering in my chest. It was beating lightly but extremely fast like a hummingbird, and I had no idea what was going on. It stopped after a few minutes, and later when I described it to my doctor, she told me that it was nothing to worry about. This would go on to happen to me fairly regularly, maybe once every six months, and I always brushed it off. In my late 20s, it started happening more frequently, and for much longer periods. I would go on to learn that this was SVT. We'll cover this more in the section on SVT.

Concurrently in my mid-20s, I started having occasional palpitations, which I would later learn were PACs and PVCs. These gave me the feeling that my heart was stopping and restarting, but they were usually sporadic and isolated, occasionally occurring in longer strings. While SVT is a much scarier condition where it sometimes feels like your heart is going to explode out of your chest, the ectopic beats are simply extremely annoying. If SVT is a thunderstorm, ectopics are a light rain, but they seem to taunt you, whispering something like "you're weak" with every skipped beat. Luckily, as I have discovered over the past year, there are ways to mitigate this annoying physical phenomenon, and even get rid of them for good, if you are disciplined.

Part I: PACs and PVCs

PACs and PVCs are both forms of what are known as ectopic beats. The main pacemaker of the heart is the sinoatrial node, which sends the electrical signals that travel around the heart and cause it to beat, beginning with the atria, followed by the ventricles. An ectopic beat happens when some group of cells somewhere else in the atria (in the case of PACs) or the ventricles (in the case of PVCs) "hijacks" that natural rhythm and causes a premature beat. This is usually followed by a compensatory pause, before the heart resumes its normal rhythm. I'm not going to get any more technical than that due to my aforementioned lack of a medical degree, and the fact that while the function of the heart is very interesting, that knowledge is not of much use to most people suffering from ectopic beats.

PACs and PVCs can feel similar, but for me, the PVCs have a much more violent and surprising character. PACs can be almost imperceptible, like a light pitter-pat, while PVCs feel more like you just got punched in the stomach.

Read this next part carefully because I'm going to lay

out my main theory about ectopic beats, and that is that they are not really a heart issue. As someone who has suffered from a mix of over 200 PACs and PVCs a day, and then almost completely eliminated them, I believe there is something else going on with the nervous system and muscle tension that causes this phenomenon.

Think about it: you go to the doctor complaining of palpitations, and they give you some tests. They will start with an EKG, then probably prescribe you a Holter Monitor (basically an EKG that you wear for 24 hours or more), and maybe even give you an echocardiogram and/or stress echocardiogram. I had all these tests, and the echocardiograms showed that my heart was "completely normal". I imagine that most people reading this have had the same experience. Why then, if my heart is "completely normal" am I having these palpitations that no one else around me seems to ever experience?

Common Triggers of Ectopic Beats

Before we get into what I did to actually eliminate my ectopic beats, let's break down some of the advice that is commonly given to people suffering from them. Everyone seems to have slightly different triggers for what actually brings on their ectopics, but some of the most commonly blamed culprits include:

•**Stress.** Stress seems to make people have more heart palpitations. I think most sufferers would say that this is certainly true, but why? Everyone has stress, right? Why do tons of people who have way more anxiety and stress than me seem to not have heart palpitations? Well, people react to and hold onto stress differently. I believe that stress leading to muscle tension in certain areas, and overactive sympathetic nervous system function, causes ectopic beats. We will talk about how to solve those problems soon.

•**Caffeine.** Certain people are more sensitive to caffeine than others, and in some people it can trigger ectopic beats. But why? Once again, I believe it's because caffeine can lead to muscle tension and an overactive sympathetic nervous system.

•**Alcohol.** This is an interesting one. I believe that alcohol can be a trigger for palpitations, but it does so by acting as a diuretic and dehydrating you. Dehydration is another huge factor in ectopic beats, at least for me. If I drink plenty of water with an alcoholic beverage or two, I'm completely fine, but your mileage may vary.

•**Eating a large meal.** This gets even more interesting. Eating a large meal used to be a big trigger for me, and it's part of what contributes to a condition called "holiday heart" where even people who don't normally experience palpitations will have them after partaking in large amounts of food and alcohol. e.g. at Thanksgiving or other holidays.

The mechanism for why having a very full stomach would cause ectopic beats is a little unclear. One theory is that it has to do with a nerve connection between the stomach and the heart, specifically the vagus nerve which regulates the "rest and digest" response and also is a big player in heart rate. Personally I think it has more to do with 1) dehydration again, this time from high-sodium food, and 2) the physical position of your stomach in relation to the heart and diaphragm. Having a very full stomach pushes up on the diaphragm, making it harder to take a deep breath, and deep breathing is extremely important in mitigating ectopics.

If you have hiatal hernia and/or acid reflux, it's also possible that inflammation from the stomach acid is spreading from the esophagus to the adjacent heart.

•**Bending over.** This is a somewhat lesser-known one, but it was a very reliable trigger for me. Bending at the waist to pick something up off the floor would reliably cause a big PVC or two. Now that gets you scratching your head. Is it due to a change in blood flow? Possibly, but I'm inclined to believe that it's due to compression of the stomach and solar plexus area, which contains a large mass of sensitive nerves, many of which connect to the heart. I will discuss this more soon.

•**Lying down.** Many people report that lying down in certain positions can bring on their ectopic beats, which can even interfere with sleeping. This was never a huge problem for me, but it's likely due to the fact that the position of your heart and the blood flow in your body are changing, as well as your breathing.

•**Exercise.** It can be scary when you experience ectopics while exercising, because your heart rate and systolic blood pressure are elevated, which can make the palpitations feel more dramatic. Exercising makes your heart work harder, so if you don't exercise regularly and your heart is already feeling "irritable", it can lead to ectopics. This is ironic because I found exercise to be one of the keys to eliminating my palpitations! You just have to stick with it, which (again) we'll talk about later when I get to what actually worked for me.

•**Taking a deep breath.** This is another one that falls under the "solutions" category, but if you're not used to deep breathing, the physical squeeze that your heart gets from taking a deep breath can trigger ectopics. I think this is one of the reasons why I went so many years without breathing properly, and effectively holding my breath or breathing shallowly most of the time.

What DIDN'T Work

Let's break down a list of some of the things that are commonly recommended as remedies for ectopic beats that did not work for me at all. Some of these came by way of doctors, and some were found online.

•**Ignoring them.** The first time I wore a 24-hour

Holter Monitor, my doctor informed me that I had about 150+ PACs and PVCs throughout the day. This was nothing, he told me, they are completely benign, just don't worry about them. I wouldn't say I was worried about them, per se, and I do believe that they are totally harmless. I also understand that some people have thousands a day. However, I think it's important to listen to your body, and the ectopic beats are a tiny signal that something might be wrong. Maybe not even wrong, but off. Something is not quite right, and your body is trying to tell you that you are not quite at your best. As harmless as they may be, it became impossible to ignore them even if I wanted to.

•**Supplements.** This is where you and your wallet can get into a lot of trouble. Part of why I'm writing this book is to tell you that you don't need to spend a dime to get rid of your ectopic beats! First of all, it is important to get your blood work done. Find out your electrolyte levels and see if you are deficient in anything like potassium, magnesium, or iron. I tried taking a lot of different supplements for significant periods of time based on internet anecdotes, and none of them made a bit of difference. A short list of these include: magnesium, iron, l-carnitine, B vitamins, fish oil, vitamin D and CoQ10.

•**Dietary changes.** It's easy to get caught up in hysteria around your diet and trying to figure out if certain foods aggravate your ectopic beats. I do believe that certain foods can bring on palpitations, but eliminating those foods won't address their underlying cause. Some of my suspected dietary triggers were peanut butter, chocolate and and MSG. For a while I did eliminate those foods, but it still didn't cure my ectopic beats because my diet was not the underlying cause. I experimented with different dietary changes like going low carb, low sodium or eliminating grains, but I would recommend just eating a normal, balanced, nutritious diet. Now I can eat anything I want to and not worry about palpitations.

•**Beta blockers.** In November of 2016 I was prescribed Atenolol, a long-acting beta blocker, for my SVT. It was quite effective for its intended purpose, which I will talk more about in the SVT section, but I could tell immediately that it wasn't going to do any good for my ectopic beats. The first time I took it, I felt relief for the slowing effect it had on my heart rate and the lessening of anxiety, but the PVCs and PACs were the same or even worse. More evidence, in my mind, that ectopic beats don't have much to do with your overall heart health in the traditional sense. Over time, it got even worse, until after a year of taking even a very low dose (half of a 25mg pill every day), the ectopics became more out of control than ever before. It wasn't until I was satisfied that my SVT was surgically eliminated, and I stopped taking the Atenolol and started an exercise regime, that I began to get a handle on my ectopic beats. This leads us right into the next section.

What WORKED

So here we go, I'm going to talk about how I cured my ectopic beats. I don't know if these techniques will work for everyone, but everything I'm going to lay out here is safe and completely free, so I feel no hesitation in recommending them to any healthy individual.

•**Exercise.** This is probably the biggest one, but it's also not the whole picture. Due to dealing with SVT for years, I got to the point where I was terrified of exercise, even walking up a flight of stairs. I've always maintained a healthy body weight, thanks mostly to genetic good fortune, and I have a job where I'm on my feet all day, so I also didn't really feel like I needed to exercise. When I did exercise, even if an attack of SVT didn't come on, I would often experience ectopic beats either during or after.

As I mentioned above, I (spoiler alert) had a surgical ablation for my SVT. I continued taking Atenolol for a few months after the procedure, until it finally dawned on me that it had actually worked and I was free of SVT. During this time, though, the PACs and PVCs continued to worsen, until I made the step really begin exercising.

So what form of exercise to do? For me, the most effective thing has been relatively short but medium-high intensity aerobic/cardiovascular workouts. I started by simply walking up a single flight of stairs 35 or 40 times, because that was also a way of conquering a specific fear that I had. I worked my way up to running the stairs, 50 or 60 times up and down. This takes me about 15 minutes, and if I do that three to four times a week, I see a dramatic reduction in my ectopic beats.

Note that the first few times I practiced this workout, my ectopics actually got worse, during the exercise and then for about an hour afterwards. Don't be alarmed if this happens to you. I just kept doing it, and after a couple of weeks, I started to notice dramatic results.

Why does exercise work? I think it's more complex than simply improving your overall cardiovascular fitness, though that can't hurt at all either. Beta blockers can simulate being in good cardiovascular shape by reducing your heart rate and blood pressure, and those did nothing for my ectopics. I think the real benefit of exercise is the breath, which is why I like moderate to high intensity workouts. Here is where things get murky because I don't think anyone really knows the exact mechanism that is at work here, but the lungs and the heart are undoubtedly closely connected. I believe that the very deep and rapid breathing during intense exercise calms the sympathetic nervous system, which ultimately is at the root of why we experience ectopics.

Of course, talk to your doctor before starting a new exercise program.

•**Hydration.** Again, I'm not sure exactly why, but for me, hydration is a key part in preventing ectopic beats. Drink water throughout the day, especially if you ingest any diuretic substance, and if you're like me, you're likely to see a reduction in palpitations.

•**Deep breathing.** Even when you're not exercising, you can practice deep breathing. This will effectively calm your sympathetic nervous system, and probably reduce palpitations. Breathe deeply and slowly in and out through your nose and inhale into your stomach. This works best in combination with muscle relaxation.

•**Muscle relaxation.** This is a big one. I once asked my primary care doctor if she thought that muscle tension in my chest, back and stomach could be contributing to my PACs and PVCs. She said no, and I think she was wrong. Have you ever noticed that thinking and obsessing about your palpitations actually makes them worse? I certainly did. I think this is because when we dwell on negative emotions and anxiety, we become tense, and there are a few areas in particular that can be problematic. Fear sends a message to our muscles to tense up, and if we don't let go of that tension, it can create a feedback loop telling our body that there is danger or something wrong.

When someone tells you to relax, it can be easier said than done, and I think trying to relax the mind is the wrong place to start. If you can actually physically relax and stretch out the muscles in places where you hold onto fear and anxiety, it will produce an unexpected feeling of euphoria that instantly puts your mind more at ease. It will put an end to the feedback loop between mind and body saying that there is something wrong, which should in turn relax the sympathetic nervous system and reduce your palpitations.

For me, the most important area to relax is the upper abdominal muscles, just below the sternum. I came to realize that I was walking around with these muscles tense almost 100% of the time, to the point that I was pushing in my abdomen and (I think) irritating nerves in my solar plexus area. If I consciously relax these muscles, it helps tremendously, and even better is to stretch them out. Grab onto something high up, like the top of a door, and put yourself in a semi-suspended state where you can really feel the upper abdominal muscles on both sides getting a good stretch, all the way up to the top. After I do this, it's hard to stop myself from laughing in relief, and it feels like tension and fear are literally leaving my body.

Another area of tension for me is the shoulders and

mid back, and this is greatly exacerbated by the use of a smart phone. Ever wonder why the number of people complaining of ectopic beats seems to be on the rise? I think it could have a lot to do with everyone being hunched over their cell phones, creating significant muscle tension. Even sitting here typing on the computer feels like an unnatural act, and I'll certainly do some stretching after I get up. I think many people who are anxious or worried keep their shoulders tense and slightly elevated. Stand with your back straight, arms straight down and push your hands down towards the floor as far as you can for a few seconds at a time, without changing posture. Your shoulders will come down and feel much more relaxed. For the mid to upper back, pretend like you are giving yourself a really strong hug, and twist from side to side until you can feel the muscles adjacent to your spine stretching.

•**Ridiculously deep breathing.** This is a term I've coined, and in my mind I refer to it as 'RDB' for short. This takes deep breathing to a whole new level, but it really helps for relaxation and relief of muscle tension. It's a bit hard to describe, but imagine taking the deepest breath you could take, then taking it even deeper. For this

I am mostly breathing into my chest rather than pushing down into my stomach. Treat it as though you are trying as hard as you can to expand your rib cage, by pushing out hard with your lungs. You can hold this and keep pushing outwards for several seconds. Pay special attention to expanding your chest on the left side closest to your heart. As someone who has probably been a shallow breather all my life, this does wonders, and even helps stretch out and relax the muscles in my back and shoulders. As with all of these techniques, the bonus is that it just feels good!

So there you have it. I hope this section was clear in laying out my ideas about what causes ectopic beats, and what you can do to prevent and eliminate them. Hopefully it gave you some actionable techniques that you can use in your everyday life.

Part II: SVT

While the story of conquering my PACs and PVCs was all about looking within myself to understand where I was holding onto tension and fear, my journey with SVT was much more about interacting with and navigating the medical establishment. It took me some time to get there, though. I mentioned in the introduction that I first experienced SVT when I was 17 years old in 2003, long before I learned what it was or anything about it. For most of the next 13 years, it was a rare occurrence, with an episode coming on maybe every six months to a year. I was able to shrug it off as a strange anomaly that always went back to normal within a few minutes. As the years went on, it started to become a little more scary. It still wasn't happening every day or even every month, but the episodes were lasting longer, and the realization that this wasn't just going to "go away", along with a bit of anxiety about when it would happen again, started to come on my radar.

If you're reading this, I assume you probably know what SVT feels like. Maybe you've been diagnosed with it, or maybe you just suspect you have it by comparing notes with fellow sufferers. When you feel it coming on, you immediately think "oh no, here it goes again". In my case it was always a sudden onset, where my heart would accelerate to three or four times its normal rate. I would feel it beating out of my chest and wonder ,"When will it stop? Am I going to die this time?". When it happened during exercise it would be particularly scary, as the beating would be even more violent and rapid.

In 2015, I had a couple of particularly scary episodes within a couple of months of each other. One happened while I was shoveling snow, and I felt like I was going to pass out. The other was while I was giving a presentation at a trade show, and it lasted for a total of about an hour and a half. It still somehow did not quite dawn on me that this could be something serious, and I was just glad when an episode was over.

As far as what triggered my SVT, it became clear that my ectopic heart beats (PACs and PVCs), which had started increasing in frequency, were a major contributor. Other things that seemed to be able to bring it on were sudden bumps and jolts to my body, but still it was relatively infrequent.

In February of 2016, we had an unseasonably warm day and my wife and I decided to go for a hike. At this point, she was faintly aware of the fact that this weird heart thing happened to me sometimes, but had never witnessed it first hand. We hiked down a big hill and then back up. Just as we reached the top of the hill, boom, the SVT kicked in. I waited for it to go away, but it showed no signs of doing so. I managed to get to the car, and eventually just decided to drive home. After we got home, it kept on going for the rest of afternoon as I tried to rest and relax. When it finally stopped, it had been over three and a half hours. At this point, you may think that going to the hospital would have been wise, and you'd probably be right. But no, I toughed it out and carried on.

June 2016, our wedding anniversary. We had a fantastic meal and a glass of wine, but on the way back to the car, here it comes again. This time it went away after an hour, but I had simply had enough. It was finally time to go see a doctor and figure out what exactly was going on. The problem was, though, that SVT is a very tricky thing to catch on an EKG. Even though the anxiety about my condition had finally caught up to me, which in turn caused my episodes to become more frequent over the next few months, we simply could not get a tracing of it while it was actually going on. Holter Monitors and EKGs all showed nothing but ectopic beats here and there, and I was still in the dark about what this condition was even called.

Due to seemingly interminable delays in scheduling appointments, I did not see my first cardiologist until November of 2016. After a relatively short office visit, I came away with appointments for an echocardiogram and a stress echo, as well as a bit more knowledge about this condition, that my cardiologist believed was the "God-given" gift known as supraventricular tachycardia, SVT. He explained to me there is a normal pathway for how electrical impulses move throughout the heart, and that some people randomly develop an extra pathway, which creates a smaller circuit, leading to episodes of extremely fast heart rate. Oh, and I came away with one other thing. I asked if there was any sort of prescription he could write that would help with the anxiety of this condition, and on the way home I stopped at the pharmacy and picked up my first bottle of the beta blocker atenolol.

Atenolol - A Game Changer

I waited until the next morning to take my first 25mg dose of atenolol. As soon as it hit my system, I began to feel "normal" again. I told my wife that I felt like I had felt before all this had hit the fan, before the anxiety of an unknown and worsening heart condition at the age of 30 had overtaken me. My heart rate slowed down to the point where it felt like an attack of SVT was almost impossible, and I actually felt relaxed for the first time in months. It gave me some breathing room to step back and actually reflect on what was happening, and it felt like a miracle drug.

But What if I Could do Better?

I continued taking the atenolol for a few weeks, and it worked quite well. Not perfectly, though. I still had some brief episodes of SVT while I was on it, and I even began to resent the suffocating "downer" effect that it had on me.

I started asking myself, "Do I want to be on this for the rest of my life?". My tolerance for SVT had become so low that even a few seconds of it would throw me into a funk. I knew that surgical ablation could be an option for SVT, but I also knew that without getting an official EKG tracing of what was going on with my heart, I couldn't even get in the door to talk to a surgeon. So one evening I decided to put my foot down and commit to working towards getting the surgery.

The first step was, of course, that EKG. I went to see my cardiologist, and in January I received an event monitor in the mail, that I would wear for 21 days in an effort to capture the whatever-it-was. This meant going off the atenolol completely, strapping several electrodes to my chest daily, and carrying around a PDA device that would transmit my EKG tracing to the company when I was having an episode.

I have to admit, trying to trigger my arrhythmia was sort of fun. I got to do all the things that my cardiologist had warned me against: drinking alcohol and caffeine, exercising, not taking the atenolol, eating foods that I thought were triggers, even taking some cold medicine that

I thought had brought on an episode once. All with the electrodes stuck to my chest, waiting to pick up any abnormalities. Once I drank a glass of red wine, took the cold medicine, and ran up and down the stairs for half an hour. Surprisingly, nothing happened. It seemed to be much harder to trigger it when I was actually trying to, than when I was anxiously dreading an episode. The cruel tricks that our bodies play on us sometimes.

It took 10 or 11 days before I was actually able to trigger an episode of my arrhythmia. It took a large cup of black coffee and a good session of snow shoveling, and I felt that old familiar feeling come back. I pulled out the PDA, hit "send" and hoped it was coming through nice and clear to the monitoring company in Texas. I popped an atenolol, and thankfully was back to normal in about 15 minutes. For the first time ever with an episode of SVT, I was feeling elated. "I got it!", I told my wife. This was a big step toward doing something to permanently eliminate this scary, condition that I had been dealing with off and on for 13 years.

At my next appointment with my cardiologist, he informed me that the tracing came through beautifully. It was in fact SVT, and it clocked in at a nice, clean 210 beats per minute. We were ready to take the next step.

Exploring Surgical Ablation

My cardiologist referred me to a surgeon in a nearby city, one of the best in the country, he informed me, with six other surgeons training in performing this procedure under him. Naturally, I had done some searching for information on the internet, and the numbers I was seeing didn't look too great. Most of the websites I looked at were estimating the effectiveness of surgical ablation for SVT at around 50-70%, and the cost at $35,000 or more. Many people reported having to go back for another round of the procedure because their SVT came back, though sometimes it was reduced to shorter episodes. However, based on the assurances of my cardiologist that this particular surgeon had a greater than 90% success rate, I was feeling positive as I drove up for my first consultation.

After arriving at the hospital, I first spoke with a nurse practitioner who described what would be involved with the procedure, as well as the risks. During an ablation, catheters are inserted into the femoral artery by way of a very small incision in the groin area, and then make their way to the heart. The ultimate goal is to use a catheter with a heated tip to burn the small part of the heart tissue that is conducting electricity improperly. The heart is supposed to be covered with a sort of electrically resistant tissue, so that the electrical impulses only travel on the proper pathway to make the heart beat normally. In people with SVT, as it was described to me, there is a small gap or space in that tissue that can hijack the electrical signal, leading to a sort of "short circuit". During the ablation, the burning of that area creates scar tissue which effectively re-insulates it.

An ablation can be a fairly long procedure (ask me how I know), because they need to begin by mapping out where exactly the tissue is that needs to be burned. It can be in a number of different areas in the left or right atrium, some of which are quite sensitive and carry a higher risk of complications. If the area is too close to the sinoatrial node, there is a risk of damaging the heart's main pacemaker and having to implant an artificial one. Without knowing exactly where the burn would take place, they assigned an overall probably of that happening at about 1%, with the risk of death being much less than 1%. There are different sub-categories of SVT, depending on where the problem area is located. The main ones are Atrioventricular Node Re-Entrant Tachycardia (AVNRT) and Atrioventricular Reciprocating Tachycardia (AVRT).

After seeing the nurse practitioner, I spoke with the surgeon. He reiterated the details and the risks, but I had already made up my mind. We scheduled a date for the surgery, only a few weeks away. When you feel like you can't fully live your life in your current state, you're much more likely to be willing to roll the dice on a risk-reward proposition.

The Procedure

I arrived at the hospital at the appointed time, which was quite early in the morning on April 18, 2017. A nurse had the unenviable job of completely shaving my upper body, and then I met with the surgeon (actually two of them - he had a colleague to assist in the procedure). Everyone seemed upbeat and I was ready to put my life in their capable hands.

Lying on the operating table, I began to feel the effects of the anesthesia, propofol and fentanyl if I remember correctly. Three small punctures were made in my groin to allow the catheters to enter my femoral artery. I don't pretend to know the actual techniques used, but the first part of the procedure is referred to as "mapping", where they locate the area in the heart that needs to be cauterized. In order to do this, they need to actually observe the arrhythmia in action, which is why they tell you to stop using any beta blockers several days before the procedure.

Because of the fact that it's very difficult to trigger any form of tachycardia when you're under general anesthetic, they will adjust your level of sedation higher and lower depending on what part of the procedure they're doing. During the mapping, the surgeons need to have total control of your heart, and can use substances or "pacing" to accelerate it to the point where it goes into arrhythmia. This also means that you need to be at least partially awake because the anesthesia can suppress tachycardia, and I can very vividly remember this part of the procedure. It was definitely painful and unpleasant, but I was still out of it enough to not care too much.

I certainly didn't remember the whole procedure, because when I woke up I had the feeling that the whole thing had lasted only about half an hour. In reality, it was closer to three and a half hours. The surgeon came to see me and let me know that he thought the operation had been a success. The site that needed to be cauterized turned out to be fairly close to the sinoatrial node, but with enough distance that the procedure could be safely completed. He also told me for the first time exactly what variety of SVT I had - it turned out to be the more rare "atypical AVNRT", which is the case for only a small percentage of people with SVT. Lucky me!

After the Ablation

My trusty surgeon informed me that there is a healing period after this procedure, both for the incision in my groin and for the heart. He told me that my PACs and PVCs might actually increase for a week or two, but as long as I didn't have any SVT I knew I would be fine. He also told me to keep taking the atenolol for a while, but that I could get off it after a few months.

I felt like I made a good recovery in the following days, and was back to all my normal activities within a week. The thing about this procedure though, is that it takes quite a while to prove to yourself that it really worked. I could easily go a couple of months without having any SVT normally, especially while taking the atenolol, so how did I know if I just happened to not have it for a while? Over the last 15 months since I had the procedure as of this writing, I have had a few sporadic instances of very short bits of SVT, lasting no more than a couple of seconds or 4-5 beats. To me, this is the exception that proves the rule. Those are moments where I WOULD have launched into full-blown SVT, possibly for hours, but instead it's gone in the blink of an eye. It just proves to me that the surgeons didn't go too far with the burn, for which I am very grateful.

At this point, I consider myself completely cured of SVT, and I feel that making the decision to have the surgery was one of the best decisions of my life. I'm in awe at the skill of my surgeons and eternally grateful to them. I hope that whoever is reading this who is on the fence about how to proceed with treating their SVT, has gained some knowledge or insight from this section. Whether the treatment be pharmaceutical or surgical, I hope that my story has helped to clear up some of the mystery around this condition and its treatment.